Fabián Arias
Cristian Lagla
Bryan Vaca

PERIPHERAL ARTERIAL DISEASE

Fabián Arias
Cristian Lagla
Bryan Vaca

PERIPHERAL ARTERIAL DISEASE

DIAGNOSIS AND TREATMENT

ScienciaScripts

Imprint
Any brand names and product names mentioned in this book are subject to trademark, brand or patent protection and are trademarks or registered trademarks of their respective holders. The use of brand names, product names, common names, trade names, product descriptions etc. even without a particular marking in this work is in no way to be construed to mean that such names may be regarded as unrestricted in respect of trademark and brand protection legislation and could thus be used by anyone.

Cover image: www.ingimage.com

This book is a translation from the original published under ISBN 978-620-2-11378-6.

Publisher:
Sciencia Scripts
is a trademark of
Dodo Books Indian Ocean Ltd. and OmniScriptum S.R.L publishing group

120 High Road, East Finchley, London, N2 9ED, United Kingdom
Str. Armeneasca 28/1, office 1, Chisinau MD-2012, Republic of Moldova, Europe
Printed at: see last page
ISBN: 978-620-5-74697-4

PERIPHERAL ARTERIAL DISEASE - DIAGNOSIS AND TREATMENT

Introduction

Peripheral arterial disease is a condition characterised by a decrease in arterial blood flow posterior to the aortic arch, secondary to an obstructive mechanism, either intrinsic or extrinsic, and is mainly caused by atherosclerosis, which is caused by an abnormal accumulation of lipoprotein particles (LDL) and fibrous tissue between the intimal and muscular layer of the arterial wall. (1) Its forms of presentation include intermittent claudication, pain at rest (these with trophic changes due to ischaemia such as ulceration) and critical lower limb ischaemia. Many studies have shown a direct association with increased cardiovascular morbidity and mortality and the development of peripheral arterial disease (1,2). An ankle-brachial index (ABI) ≤ 0.90 is associated with more than doubled rates of coronary events, CV event mortality and total mortality at 10 years. After 5 years, 20% of patients with intermittent claudication (IC) develop myocardial infarction (MI) or stroke and mortality is 10-15%. Early diagnosis and proper management are of paramount importance to minimise the above complications (1,3).

<u>**Pathophysiology**</u>

Abnormal accumulation of lipids and fibrous tissue beneath the vascular intima can lead to narrowing of the vessel lumen; multiple factors contribute to the pathogenesis of atherosclerosis, including endothelial dysfunction, dyslipidaemia, inflammatory and immunological factors and cigarette smoking (1).

The endothelium represents a biological interface between the blood and the rest of the tissues, and has properties such as regulation of tone, growth and haemostasis. When endothelial dysfunction occurs, nitric oxide release is lost, decreasing its anti-inflammatory and vasodilatory action. Simultaneously, while an inflammatory process is taking place, LDL accumulation occurs in the arterial wall and endothelial cells express several adhesion molecules (VCAM-1, adhesins), which allow leukocyte adhesion with subsequent accumulation of inflammatory macrophages. (1,2) These activated leukocytes release proteolytic enzymes and a variety of peptide growth factors and cytokines that degrade matrix proteins and stimulate smooth muscle cells, endothelial cells and macrophages. Foam cells then aggregate as an effect of macrophage deposition of oxidised LDL. Subsequently, calcium accumulates in the atheroma with the expression of muscle cells and proteins involved in osteogenesis. Thus, deposition of these in the arteries of the lower limbs leads to progressive narrowing to form arterial insufficiency. (1,3)

Arterial obstruction by flow-limiting lesions underlies manifestations of peripheral arterial disease in the lower extremities. In a model of demand ischaemia, intermittent claudication reflects an inadequate increase in skeletal muscle perfusion during exercise.(2,3)

However, several lines of evidence indicate that the drivers of limb symptoms in peripheral arterial disease are more complex. Atherosclerotic disease occurs in the context of multiple pathological processes that interfere with exercise capacity. Potential mechanisms are detailed in Figure 1 and current evidence supporting the role of reduced blood flow, vascular dysfunction, altered muscle metabolism, altered angiogenesis and inflammatory activation in the production of limb discomfort and functional limitation is discussed in this section. (2,4)

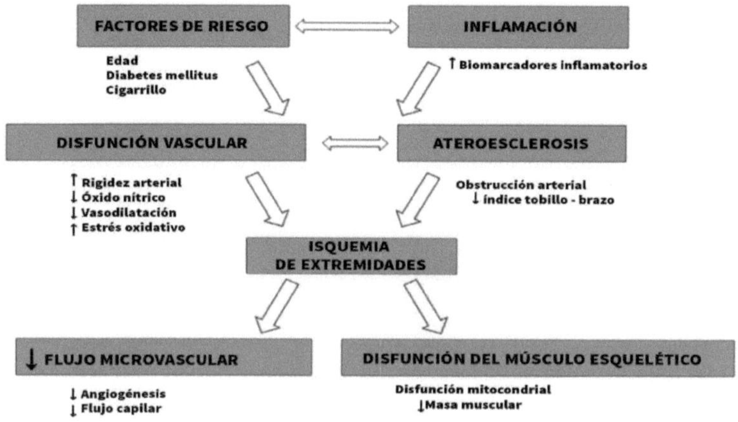

Reduced limb perfusion caused by obstructive arterial lesions

Reduced blood flow in the extremities due to atherosclerotic disease characterises peripheral arterial disease. Measurement of the ankle-arm index assesses the severity of atherosclerosis affecting blood flow between the aorta and the ankle. (1) Obstructive lesions create drops in both blood pressure and flow that add to the pressure reduction at the ankle. With exercise, flow to the lower extremity increases and magnifies the pressure drop across fixed lesions, increasing sensitivity to detect peripheral arterial disease. (2,3)

Recent studies highlight the clinical significance of an abnormal exercise ankle-arm index with an additive prognostic value for future limb revascularisation and death compared to resting ankle-arm index alone. Inadequate perfusion with exercise, which is caused by fixed lesions, is clearly a key component underlying limb symptoms in peripheral arterial disease. However, multiple studies indicate that the generation of limb ischaemia in peripheral arterial disease has multiple determinants. (1,4)

The anatomical severity of the obstruction is an imprecise predictor of clinical status and course. It is well established that patients with peripheral arterial disease have an impaired functional status compared to individuals with a normal ankle-arm index. However, some studies have shown a modest correlation between ankle-arm index and walking ability and other studies have found no association between ankle-arm index and the magnitude of functional limitation. (1,4)

Limb blood flow, assessed by other techniques, has shown inconsistent associations with functional measures. Measurement of calf blood flow based on magnetic resonance imaging was moderately related to distance travelled, but plethysmography-based calf blood flow showed no association with treadmill walking or changes in walking time. (1,4)

Prospective studies confirm that people with an abnormal ankle-arm index have a greater decline in walking ability at 2-year follow-up. However, the association between the magnitude of the reduction in ankle-arm index and functional outcomes is less clear. Taken together, the available evidence indicates that anatomical disease does not completely govern the clinical status of patients with peripheral arterial disease. (1,4)

Vascular dysfunction in peripheral arterial disease

Arterial insufficiency in peripheral arterial disease reflects both fixed and dynamic reductions in blood flow. A healthy vascular endothelium produces several vasodilatory substances, including nitric oxide, which has pluripotent vascular benefits, such as inhibiting platelets, reducing smooth muscle proliferation, preventing leukocyte adhesion and promoting angiogenesis. Decreased nitric oxide bioactivity in the leg prevents increased blood flow with exercise. Vascular dysfunction may also exacerbate the vasoconstrictor effects of catecholamines and limit flow-mediated dilation. (2,4)

Together, the effects of abnormal endothelial function may worsen clinical symptoms in peripheral arterial disease. Several studies have described the clinical relevance of endothelial dysfunction in peripheral arterial disease. Measures of endothelium-dependent vasodilator function, including brachial artery flow-mediated dilatation and acetylcholine-induced vasodilatation, are lower in patients with peripheral arterial disease. Both conduit and microvascular endothelial function were assessed in 1,320 subjects, including 377 with peripheral artery disease, and compared with patients with coronary artery disease; patients with peripheral artery disease had more severe impairment of multiple metrics of vasodilator function. The presence of endothelial dysfunction in patients with peripheral arterial disease is consistent with systemic impairment of vascular function.(3,4)

Impaired hyperemic blood flow response is associated with functional impairment in peripheral arterial disease. There is evidence linking increased brachial flow-mediated dilation with increased physical activity in daily life in patients with peripheral arterial disease. Recent studies linked impaired brachial flow-mediated dilation with reduced self-reported walking ability and a 6-minute walk test.(3,4)

Interestingly, patients with peripheral arterial disease have decreased flow-mediated dilatation of the superficial femoral artery associated with injury severity. Measures of arterial stiffness, including higher pulse pressure and augmentation index, are also associated with reduced walking time in patients with peripheral arterial disease. Endothelial dysfunction measured by brachial flow-mediated dilation and reactive hyperemia predicts an increased risk of events after vascular surgery. Whether endothelial dysfunction predicts progressive functional deterioration has not been evaluated.(4,5)

Impaired angiogenesis and reduced microcirculatory flow

Chronic limb ischaemia initiates several vascular structural adaptations. The insufficient blood supply produced by arterial ischaemia induces a complex vascular growth programme. Multiple factors that regulate angiogenesis have been identified in animal models, including vascular endothelial growth factor (VEGF), fibroblast growth factor, hepatocyte growth factor and hypoxia-inducible factor 1-α. In addition, specific bone marrow-derived cells can target regions of ischaemia and promote vessel regeneration. (3,5,8) Genetic regulators, including microRNA, are also important for angiogenesis. MicroRNA shows lower expression in animals genetically predisposed to severe clinical phenotypes, such as hind paw ischaemia. In animal models, there is abundant evidence that therapies that stimulate angiogenesis increase skeletal muscle perfusion and restore functional status.(3,4,6)

In patients with peripheral arterial disease, inadequate angiogenesis and collateral formation may enhance limb ischaemia and serve as a mechanism driving functional impairment. One study found that lower capillary density in patients with peripheral arterial disease, assessed by skeletal muscle biopsy, was associated with reduced functional measures, including maximal walking time. Similarly, imaging studies using MRI or contrast-enhanced ultrasound have demonstrated lower microvascular flow in the calf musculature in patients with peripheral arterial disease.(2,7)

Exercise blood flow measured by contrast ultrasound was related to claudication time in a treadmill test. In addition, reduced skeletal muscle blood flow measured by MRI during exercise was associated with reduced 6-minute walk time. Taken together, the clinical research evidence supports the concept that microcirculatory dysfunction affects limb function in patients with peripheral arterial disease and that increasing calf blood flow may be a therapeutic avenue. Therefore, proangiogenic therapy approaches to treat peripheral arterial disease have been used in many studies of growth factor and cell-based therapies.(2,4,5)

As recently reviewed, these clinical trials have failed to convincingly demonstrate a reduction in limb symptoms, including pain and wound healing. There are a number of possible explanations for the disappointment with proangiogenic interventions in patients with peripheral arterial disease. Translational studies emphasise the relevance of systemic disease and risk factors for impaired angiogenesis in clinical peripheral arterial disease. Paradoxically, patients with peripheral arterial disease have higher levels of VEGF-A, a key promoter of angiogenesis. (3,6,7)

A recent study found evidence that an anti-angiogenic isoform of VEGF, VEGF-165b, is upregulated in both preclinical models and patients with PAD. The enhanced expression of anti-angiogenic VEGF is driven by the proinflammatory Wnt5a/JNK pathway, which is activated by obesity. Therefore, metabolic dysfunction may mediate inappropriate angiogenesis in peripheral arterial disease by generating anti-angiogenic factors and complicating responses to therapies aimed at stimulating angiogenesis. (3,5)

Resolvin D2, an anti-inflammatory regulator of tissue repair responses, is important both in models of hind paw ischaemia and in patients with peripheral arterial disease. Resolvin D2 treatment improves arteriogenesis and reduces inflammation, even in diabetic animals. Therefore, the next generation of proangiogenic therapies may require evaluation in animal models with metabolic dysfunction and targeting both inflammation and vascular growth.(4,5)

Skeletal muscle disorders and mitochondrial dysfunction

Repeated episodes of ischaemia have deleterious effects on the skeletal musculature of the limbs. The altered metabolic and structural properties of skeletal muscle magnify ischaemia-induced functional impairment. Computed tomography imaging studies demonstrate that patients with peripheral arterial disease have a reduced calf muscle area that is not fully explained by inactivity. In addition, skeletal muscle shows reduced density and increased fat content, which may limit muscle function. On muscle biopsy, there is increased muscle cell apoptosis and reduced fibre type content, which may interfere with performance (2,4).

Ischaemia also impairs peripheral nerve function, with evidence of impaired nerve conduction in patients with severe peripheral arterial disease. Mitochondrial dysfunction contributes to impaired skeletal muscle metabolism in peripheral arterial disease. Both circulating and muscle levels of oxidative phosphorylation intermediates, including acylcarnitines, are higher in peripheral arterial disease, suggesting reduced mitochondrial metabolism. In muscle tissue, mitochondrial mass is higher; however, there is reduced activity of several mitochondrial complexes that prevent ATP generation and enhance the production of reactive oxygen species. Impaired mitochondrial function restricts oxygen utilisation and may also promote endothelial dysfunction as mitochondrial-derived oxidants reduce nitric oxide bioactivity (2,4,5).

Muscle fibre degeneration is associated with evidence of oxidative stress, including carbonyl groups and 4-hydroxy-2-nonenal adducts, protein modifications produced by reactive oxygen species. Mitochondrial function is also important in angiogenesis, in line with the notion of coupling of muscle and vascular parameters. In models of hind paw ischaemia, peroxisome proliferator-activated receptor γ coactivator 1α (PGC 1α), a key regulator of mitochondrial biogenesis, promotes vascular regeneration.(3,5)

Altered muscle metabolism also reflects reduced nutrient absorption related to systemic metabolic disorders in patients with peripheral arterial disease. Patients with peripheral arterial disease show insulin resistance and insulin resistance predicts an increased risk of developing clinical peripheral arterial disease. By assessing skeletal muscle glucose uptake with PET, peripheral arterial disease patients with intermittent claudication have been shown to have insulin resistance in calf muscles. (2,5) Further studies are needed to link muscle insulin resistance to functional parameters in peripheral arterial disease and to determine whether interventions to promote insulin sensitivity will reduce limb symptoms.

Skeletal muscle dysfunction, including mitochondrial abnormalities, affects walking ability in peripheral arterial disease. Both decreased calf muscle content and altered fibre type are associated with reduced functional parameters. (1,5) Importantly, mitochondrial dysfunction assessed by MR spectroscopy to evaluate phosphocreatine recovery is associated with reduced treadmill walking time. Patients with peripheral arterial disease with higher amounts of muscle acylcarnitine accumulation have higher degrees of exercise limitation. Evidence of myofibre damage is associated with both reduced walking distance and muscle strength in patients with claudication. In addition, altered regulation of a cytoskeletal protein, desmin, is associated with reduced mitochondrial respiratory function and functional capacity in peripheral arterial disease. (4,5)

There is evidence of inadequate mitochondrial clearance through autophagy in skeletal muscle in peripheral arterial disease that is associated with gait parameters consistent with increased mitochondrial damage. Higher levels of daily activity are associated with healthy calf muscle parameters. Several aspects of skeletal muscle phenotype, including increased calf muscle fat and decreased muscle density, predicted a 2-year functional decline in a longitudinal study. (5,7)

Evidence of reduced mitochondrial biogenesis is associated with increased overall mortality, which is potentially mediated by reduced physical activity (5).

Systemic and Local Inflammation

Inflammatory activation is involved in the development of atherosclerosis and may play a role in the generation of limb symptoms. Circulating biomarkers of systemic inflammation, including C-reactive protein (CRP) and soluble intracellular adhesion molecule-1 (sICAM-1), predict an increased risk of developing clinical peripheral arterial disease. (3,6) In patients with established peripheral arterial disease, higher levels of inflammatory biomarkers are associated with both progression of lower extremity arterial obstruction and risk of cardiovascular events. Skeletal muscle ischaemia can cause local inflammation, exacerbate symptoms and alter muscle metabolism. In imaging studies, the lower calf muscle area and the higher fat content of the calf muscle were associated with systemic inflammation. Vascular inflammation also alters dynamic responses by reducing nitric oxide bioactivity, leading to a decrease in endothelium-mediated vasodilation.(5,8)

Inflammation has been associated with reduced walking ability in patients with peripheral arterial disease. Markers of vascular inflammation are associated with lower functional measures in patients with peripheral arterial disease, Wnt5a is associated with a lower ankle-arm index. In patients with peripheral arterial disease, a higher degree of daily physical activity is associated with lower levels of CRP, IL-6, fibrinogen, sICAM-1 and sVCAM-1. In prospective studies, functional decline is lower in patients with peripheral artery disease with lower CRP levels.(5,11)

<u>**Epidemiology**</u>

The global prevalence of peripheral arterial disease of the lower extremities is between 3 and 12 per cent. In 2010, 202 million people worldwide were living with peripheral arterial disease. The majority of people with peripheral artery disease (70 percent) live in low/middle-income regions of the world, including 55 million people in Southeast Asia and 46 million in the Western Pacific region, so its incidence is affected by psycho-social factors.(6,8)

In a report from the US National Health and Nutrition Examination Survey (NHANES), in which peripheral arterial disease was defined as an ankle-brachial ITB <0.9 in either leg, the prevalence of PAD among adults aged 40 years and older in the US was 4.3 per cent, corresponding to approximately 5 million people. (7) PAD is more common in older people, in people of certain ethnicities, in families with atherosclerosis and in people with risk factors for cardiovascular disease. In the NHANES study, more than 95 percent of people with peripheral arterial disease had one or more risk factors for cardiovascular disease. (8,9)

The prevalence of peripheral arterial disease is strongly related to age, increasing >10% among patients aged 60-70 years. Prevalence appears to be higher among men than among women for more severe or symptomatic disease. (7,9)

The American College of Cardiology/American Heart Association (ACC/AHA) guidelines on PAD have identified risk groups that are associated with a higher prevalence of peripheral artery disease (Table 1) and an earlier onset of symptomatic PAD. Patients in these groups should be evaluated for peripheral arterial disease (9,10).

Table 1. Patients at Increased Risk of Peripheral Artery Disease (8)

Age over 65 and,
Age 50 - 64 years, with risk factors for atherosclerosis (e.g. diabetes mellitus, history of smoking, hyperlipidaemia, hypertension) or family history of PAD.
Age less than 50 years and, diabetes mellitus and an additional risk factor for atherosclerosis.
Individuals with known atherosclerotic disease in another vascular bed (e.g., coronary, carotid, subclavian, renal or abdominal aortic aneurysm).

<u>**Risk Factors**</u>

Risk factors for the development of Peripheral Artery Disease are:

- **Age:** The prevalence of peripheral arterial disease increases progressively with age, starting after the age of 40 years. The relationship between age and PAD was established in the NHANES study (40 to 49 years - 0.9%, 50 to 59 years - 2.5%, 60 to 69 years - 4.7%, >70 years - 14.5% and >80 years - 23.2%).(11,12)

  People older than 70 years have a significantly increased risk of PAD due to age alone, while the risk for younger people is due to other factors, most commonly smoking. However, only half of older adults with PAD have symptoms of PAD in the lower extremities, often due to other comorbidities that limit mobility, such as arthritis, heart disease and lung disease.(11,13)

  Traditional risk factors for peripheral arterial disease may be absent in patients over 80 years of age, particularly those with infrapopliteal disease (10,12).

- **Sex:** The prevalence of peripheral arterial disease, whether symptomatic or asymptomatic, is higher in men than in women, mainly in younger age groups. In patients with ischaemic heart disease the ratio of men to women is between 1:1 and 2:1, this increases in some studies to at least 3:1 in more advanced stages such as critical ischaemia of the lower limbs. (10,12)

  Whether there is any effect of hormone replacement therapy in postmenopausal women on the development of peripheral arterial disease is largely unknown. A study of 847,982 postmenopausal women found that, despite a higher prevalence of several atherosclerotic risk factors among women using hormone replacement therapy, they were significantly less likely to have peripheral artery disease.(10,12)

- **Race:** The prevalence of peripheral arterial disease is higher in black individuals (prevalence of 7.8% versus 4.9% relative to non-Hispanic individuals). The NHANES study found a higher prevalence of peripheral arterial disease for African Americans (men and women), and also for Hispanic American women compared to non-Hispanic white Americans (19.2 and 19.3 percent, respectively, versus 15.6 percent). (12,14)

- **Genetic factors and family influence:** Patients with a family history of cardiovascular disease appear to be at increased risk, although the relative contributions of genetics and environmental factors are not fully elucidated, but remain an active area of research. The risk of peripheral artery disease is increased in families identified with early onset atherosclerosis, but no single genetic marker for peripheral artery disease has been identified in this population. (13,15)

Atherosclerotic disease is likely to be the result of numerous genes interacting with each other and with the environment. Studies that have investigated heritable factors in the development of peripheral artery disease include family and twin studies, analysis of variance of the ankle-arm index and genetic studies. (13,16)

The chromosome 9p21 (Chr9p21) locus, identified in 2007, was first associated with coronary artery disease and myocardial infarction, but may have a more general role in vascular pathology. Additional associations have been demonstrated for carotid artery plaque and plaque progression, peripheral arterial disease and aneurysmal disease.(14,15)

- **Smoking:** Cigarette smoking is directly linked to cardiovascular disease. The mechanism by which smoking promotes the onset or progression of atherosclerosis is unclear, but its effects include: endothelial damage, vascular smooth muscle proliferation, thrombophilia, inflammation and other metabolic abnormalities. (12,15) In the NHANES study, the risk of peripheral artery disease was increased in active smokers, while there was no association with other forms of smoking exposure (13).

In addition, there is evidence that the amount of cigarettes consumed is closely related to the occurrence of peripheral arterial disease, as the Framingham Heart Study found that the risk of developing claudication was directly related to the number of cigarettes smoked, with a 1.4-fold increase in risk for every 10 cigarettes smoked per day. (13,16) Smoking cessation decreases peripheral artery disease-related morbidity; however, the risk of progression of peripheral artery disease is significantly higher in former smokers compared to never smokers. Smoking cessation is also associated with a lower risk of graft failure after lower extremity bypass surgery. These effects are limited if the patient reduces cigarette consumption rather than quitting smoking completely. (14) Because the effect of smoking cessation on quality of life and survival is not immediately evident, patients require a high level of support to initiate and maintain smoking cessation.(14,15)

- **Diabetes:** Intermittent claudication is about twice as common among diabetic patients as among non-diabetic patients and the association between diabetes mellitus and the development of peripheral arterial disease is now well established. In addition, peripheral arterial disease in patients with diabetes is more aggressive, with early large vessel involvement along with microangiopathy.(15,17)

Patients with diabetes have advanced arterial disease at diagnosis. The NHANES study found an increased risk of peripheral arterial disease in patients with diabetes (OR 2.71, 95% CI 1.03 - 7.12). Diabetic patients with IHD have a 35% risk of sudden ischaemia and a 21% risk of major amputation, compared to 19 and 3%, respectively, in non-diabetic patients. (14,17)

- **Hypertension:** Hypertension is strongly associated with the development of atherosclerosis in men and women. It is less relevant as a risk factor than smoking and diabetes. However, the risk of developing peripheral artery disease is considered to be twice as high in patients with hypertension compared to controls. (16,17)

In the United States, the prevalence of hypertension in adults is approximately 30 per cent. However, among those with an abnormal ankle brachial index, the prevalence of hypertension in the Rotterdam Study was 60 per cent. The risk of developing symptoms of peripheral arterial disease, such as intermittent claudication, in people with hypertension was twice that of people without hypertension in the Framingham study. (18) The NHANES study found that hypertensive patients also have an even higher prevalence of asymptomatic peripheral arterial disease and, in addition, that patients with peripheral arterial disease were less likely to receive antihypertensive treatment compared to those with other forms of cardiovascular disease. The association between hypertension and peripheral arterial disease among patients older than 60 years was particularly strong in those with untreated and poorly controlled hypertension.(13,16)

- **Hyperlipidaemia:** Patients with peripheral arterial disease have higher levels of triglycerides and/or cholesterol, lipoprotein (A), apolipoprotein B compared to patients without PAD. In addition, protective lipoproteins (HDL) are decreased. (12,17) In the Framingham study, a fasting cholesterol level >7 mmol/L (270 mg/dL) was associated with a doubling of the incidence of intermittent claudication relative to a lower fasting cholesterol level; for every 40 mg/dL increase in total serum cholesterol, the odds of developing symptomatic peripheral artery disease increased by 1.2.

Treatment of hyperlipidaemia may decrease the risk of progression of peripheral arterial disease and the incidence of intermittent claudication (17).

- **Homocysteine:** This is one of the earliest markers found in relation to the onset of atherosclerosis (found to be elevated in 40% of patients with peripheral arterial disease). Homocysteine is thought to promote smooth muscle proliferation, increase arterial wall inflammation and increase levels of plasminogen activator inhibitor.

Homocysteine also interferes with nitric oxide released by endothelial cells. Excess homocysteine leads to vessel thickening, luminal stenosis and thrombus formation.(15,17)

- **Chronic Kidney Disease:** Many guidelines do not specifically identify chronic kidney disease as a risk factor for peripheral arterial disease. However, an association between peripheral arterial disease and chronic kidney disease is increasingly being recognised and reported. While an increased risk has generally been recognised for patients with severely reduced renal function, a growing number of studies have suggested an increased risk even for mildly or moderately reduced renal function. Chronic kidney disease is considered a risk equivalent of coronary heart disease. (18)

<u>**Anatomical pattern of Peripheral Arterial Disease**</u>

Atherosclerotic disease tends to be well localised within a particular vascular segment (e.g., aortoiliac, femoropopliteal, infrapopliteal), usually occurring in the proximal or middle portions of the arterial bed. Less commonly, however, the disease may occur more distally. Among the various vascular beds, atherosclerotic disease appears to follow patterns, which may also influence the natural history and progression of the disease. (20,21)

Asymptomatic: Subclinical atherosclerosis is common in asymptomatic middle-aged individuals. Most high-risk participants in the Framingham Heart Study (FHS) had subclinical disease, but extensive atherosclerosis was also observed in low-risk individuals. (21,22)

Symptomatic: in addition to the symptomatic vascular bed, patients with symptomatic disease are at risk of developing additional lesions in the same or other vascular beds, underscoring the need for continuous longitudinal follow-up. (23,24)

<u>Natural history and progression of peripheral arterial disease</u>

The clinical manifestations of peripheral arterial disease depend on the location and severity of the arterial stenosis or occlusion and range from mild limb pain with activity (e.g. claudication) to limb-threatening ischaemia, claudication) to limb-threatening ischaemia. (22) While the risk of adverse limb events is lower for asymptomatic compared to symptomatic patients, clinical manifestations may develop or progress rapidly and unpredictably in those with peripheral arterial disease who continue to smoke, or those with concomitant diabetes or renal failure. (22,25)

Asymptomatic peripheral arterial disease: Most patients with peripheral arterial disease are unaware of their disease. Less than 50 percent of patients with peripheral arterial disease and approximately 30 percent of their physicians know that peripheral arterial disease is present. (17,19)

The risk of progression from asymptomatic peripheral arterial disease to ischaemic limb symptoms requiring intervention is generally low, but may be underestimated. The progression of peripheral arterial disease as measured by changes in the ankle-arm index is similar for asymptomatic and symptomatic patients. The decline in the ankle-arm index is closely related to the initial value of the ankle-arm index at the time of initial diagnosis; a more rapid decline is observed in patients with lower initial ankle-arm index values.(18,20)

Intermittent claudication: the most common symptom among patients with peripheral arterial disease is intermittent claudication, which is muscle pain reproducible with ambulation that is relieved by rest. (21,23)

The natural history of intermittent claudication is characterised by a slow progression of symptoms. Chronic limb-threatening ischaemia rarely occurs, i.e., pain at rest, tissue loss; however, revascularisation (endovascular, surgical bypass) in patients with claudication may increase progression to chronic limb-threatening ischaemia. (20,22)

Intermittent claudication as a manifestation of peripheral arterial disease is a strong marker of generalised atherosclerosis and other cardiovascular and cerebrovascular morbidity and mortality (22,24).

In addition to high morbidity and mortality, patients with intermittent claudication have poor quality of life and high rates of depression. The adverse impact of intermittent claudication on the patient's physical and emotional well-being appears to be directly related to the ability to walk (21,22).

Chronic limb-threatening ischaemia: Chronic limb-threatening ischaemia (CLIE), formerly called critical limb ischaemia, is a clinical syndrome defined by the presence of peripheral arterial disease in combination with rest pain, gangrene or ulceration of the lower extremities lasting more than 2 weeks. Chronic limb-threatening ischaemia occurs in 1 to 2 percent of patients with symptomatic peripheral arterial disease. (20,22)

The natural history of untreated chronic limb-threatening ischaemia is difficult to elucidate, as patients undergo medical treatment to prolong survival and, in the era of endovascular therapies, many will undergo some form of intervention in an attempt to save the limb. The proportion of patients with claudication that deteriorated or progressed to chronic limb-threatening ischaemia was 21 percent (20,24).

Risk factors that increase the risk of chronic limb-threatening ischaemia include diabetes (fourfold risk), smoking (threefold risk) and hypercholesterolaemia (twofold risk) (25).

Patients with chronic limb-threatening ischaemia are at immediate risk of limb loss. Amputation rates remain high at 25 per cent and long-term survival is poor. Nearly 25 percent of patients with chronic limb-threatening ischaemia will suffer a cardiovascular death within one year of initial diagnosis. (22,25)

Limb salvage and long-term survival are significantly worse in patients with diabetes and in those who continue to smoke (24).

Clinical manifestations

Peripheral arterial disease may be asymptomatic, especially in its early stages; on the other hand, when clinical manifestations appear, they are predominantly due to progressive narrowing of the vascular lumen.   are predominantly due to progressive narrowing of the vascular lumen. Table 2 details the different manifestations of the disease (26,27).

Table 2. Symptoms related to decreased blood flow in the lower limbs (9)

Symptom	Description
Claudication	Pain in the lower extremity that starts after walking a certain distance and resolves in less than 10 minutes, allowing the patient to return to exercise.
Pain at rest	Constant discomfort or burning pain that usually occurs at rest in the forefoot and toes. The patient reports that it worsens with elevation of the limb.
Ischaemic ulceration	Formation of minor traumatic injuries that fail to heal due to reduced blood flow
Gangrene	The patient often notices areas of pallor or cyanosis when elevating the foot and redness when lowering the foot . These areas may progress to necrosis and tissue loss.

Symptoms in patients with peripheral arterial disease can be further stratified according to various classification systems that have been implemented, the most commonly used of which are the Leriche-Fontaine classification (Table 3) and the Rutherford classification (Table 4), the latter being the most recent and the one on which most current studies are based (walking impairment defining mild, moderate and severe claudication is specified by performance on a five-minute treadmill test at 2 mph at a 12 percent incline in the Rutherford classification, and as part of the Fontaine classification it is specified as 650 feet (200 metres)). These classifications have a very useful value as they confer a prognostic value and allow an indication of treatment according to the degree of this (27,29).

Table 3. Fontaine Clinical Classification - PAD (9)

Grade I	Asymptomatic. Detectable by Ankle-Brachial Index <0.9
Grade IIa	Intermittent claudication that does not limit the patient's lifestyle.
Grade IIb	Intermittent claudication that limits the patient.
Grade III	Pain or paresthesia at rest.
Grade IV	Established gangrene. Trophic lesions
Grade III and/or IV	Critical ischaemia with the risk of limb loss.

Table 4. Rutherford Clinical Classification - EAP (9)

Category	Stadium
0	Asymptomatic. Detectable by Ankle-Brachial Index <0.9
1	Mild intermittent claudication that does not limit the patient's lifestyle.
2	Moderate intermittent claudication that partially limits the patient's lifestyle.
3	Severe claudication (restricts the patient)
4	Pain or paraesthesia at rest.
5	Slight tissue loss: non-healing ulcer, focal gangrene with diffuse foot ulcer.
6	Significant loss of tissue extending above the transmetatarsal level, irrecoverable foot.

Stage I is characterised by the absence of symptoms. It includes patients with PAD, but without clinical repercussions. There are asymptomatic patients who have an extensive arterial occlusive lesion in the legs, have a sedentary lifestyle, are incapacitated by musculoskeletal or neurological disease, in these situations, patients may manifest critical ischaemia directly from an asymptomatic stage. (26,28)

Stage II is characterised by the presence of intermittent claudication. This stage is further divided into two groups: IIA refers to patients with non-disabling or long-distance claudication, while IIB refers to patients with claudication over short distances or impeding daily functionality.(27)

Intermittent claudication typical of patients with PAD is defined as the occurrence of pain in muscle masses provoked by walking and which ceases immediately after stopping exercise. It is important to note that the pain always occurs in the same muscle groups and after walking a similar distance, provided that the same slope and speed are maintained (27,29).

Stage III, representing a more advanced stage, is characterised by the presence of pain (predominant symptom) in specific muscle groups when the patient is at rest, although paresthesia/hypoesthesia in the front part of the foot and the toes are also usually present, these paresthesia at rest are usually indistinguishable from those produced by diabetic neuropathy, although the latter usually have a bilateral, symmetrical, sock-like distribution. At this stage, the patient usually presents with a cold extremity, with a variable degree of pallor. Other patients, on the other hand, present with greater ischaemia, with erythrosis of the hanging foot due to extreme cutaneous vasodilatation, known as "lobster's foot". 27,29)

The last grade of Fontaine's classification is characterised by trophic changes (ulcers) due to critical reduction of perfusion distal to the lesion, these are generally located in the extremities of the limbs, usually in the toes, or also in the malleolus or heel, these can be painless in the case of patients with concomitant diabetes and are susceptible to infection and manifest under the condition of a diabetic foot, for which the WiFi classification system is found that classifies three factors: the wound, the severity of ischaemia and the presence of infection in the foot (30):

- Wound:

    - Grade 0 - Pain at rest; no wound, no ulcer, no gangrene (30,31).
    - Grade 1: small shallow ulcer(s) on the distal part of the leg or foot, any exposed bone only limited to the distal phalanx; no gangrene, or gangrene limited to the distal toe (30,31).
    - Grade 2: deeper ulcer in the distal part of the leg or foot with exposed bone, joint or tendon, or shallow heel ulcer without calcaneal involvement; gangrenous changes confined to the toes (30,31).
    - Grade 3: extensive deep ulcer in the forefoot and/or midfoot, or full-thickness heel ulcer with or without calcaneal involvement (30,31).

- Ischaemia (note that systolic toe pressures are preferred in patients with diabetes):

    - Grade 0: ABI $\geq$0.8, ankle systolic pressure >100 mmHg, toe pressure (TP)/transcutaneous oxygen (TcPO2) $\geq$60.
    - Grade 1: ABI of 0.6 to 0.79, ankle systolic pressure of 70 to 100 mmHg, PT/TcPO2 of 40 to 59.
    - Grade 2: ABI of 0.4 to 0.59, ankle systolic pressure of 50 to 70 mmHg, PT/TcPO2 of 30 to 39.
    - Grade 3 - ABI $\leq$0.39, ankle systolic pressure <50 mmHg, PT/TcPO2 <30.

- Infection of the foot

    - Grade 0: no symptoms or signs of infection.
    - Grade 1: infection and at least two of the following are present: local swelling or induration, erythema >0.5 to $\leq$2 cm around the ulcer, local tenderness or pain,

local heat or purulent discharge. Other causes of an inflammatory skin response (e.g. gout, fracture) have been excluded (30,31).

- Grade 2: Local infection is present as defined in Grade 1 but extends >2 cm around the ulcer or involves structures deeper than the skin and subcutaneous tissues (e.g. abscess, osteomyelitis, septic arthritis, fasciitis). No clinical signs of systemic inflammatory response (30,31).

- Grade 3: local infection is present as defined for Grade 2, but clinical signs of systemic inflammatory response are manifested by two or more of the following: temperature >38 °C or <36 °C; heart rate > 90 beats per minute, respiratory rate >20 breaths per minute or PaCO2 <32 mmHg; WBC count > 12 000 or < 4 000 (cu/mm) or > 10 % immature band forms present. (30,31)

The muscle group affected will depend on the location of the occlusive lesion, although the majority present claudication in the calf muscle group, the presence of claudication in the buttocks or thighs may suggest a level of lesion in the iliac region. Table 5 shows the symptoms according to the area of arterial injury (30,32).

Table 5. Symptoms according to the area of the lesion

Injury Area	Clinical picture
Iliac aorta	Claudication in the buttock, thigh and calf. Impotence in a man (if bilateral): Leriche's disease.
Femoro popliteal	Calf claudication with/without plantar claudication
Infrapopliteal	Plantar claudication

Physical examination:

Individuals with risk factors and those with suspected symptoms of peripheral arterial disease (e.g. claudication, ischaemic pain at rest, ulcer, gangrene) should undergo cardiovascular evaluation. (31,32)

The patient's vital signs should be recorded and abnormalities noted. The patient's temperature and blood pressure at each upper extremity should be documented and the higher of the two noted for calculation of the ankle-brachial index. Fever may indicate the presence of an infected ulcer, and the presence of tachycardia and tachypnoea may support the diagnosis of a deep space infection of the foot that may not be evident on physical examination.(31,33)

Vascular examination is best performed with the patient supine on the examination table and should be performed only after the patient has rested for at least 15 minutes and warmed up if returning indoors for cold weather. Patients with advanced ischaemia who cannot tolerate having their feet elevated may be briefly placed in the supine position to examine the abdomen and femoral vessels and then seated upright for the remainder of the examination. The examination should include inspection of the skin of the extremities, examination of the abdomen, palpation of all peripheral pulses, auscultation for murmurs and neurological examination of the extremities. (31,34)

Vascular examination in patients with peripheral arterial disease commonly reveals decreased or absent pulses below the level of arterial obstruction with occasional murmurs over stenotic lesions and evidence of poor healing in the area of decreased perfusion. Other physical findings may include abnormal body habitus, changes in skin and nail colour, and abnormal venous filling time. These physical signs help determine the extent and distribution of vascular disease (32,33).

Appearance of the extremities: Changes in the appearance of the extremities depend on the duration and severity of the peripheral arterial disease. With a significant decrease in blood flow, the skin thins with functional loss of dermal appendages, which manifests as dry, shiny and hairless skin. However, one study found that lack of hair on the lower extremities is not a predictor of peripheral arterial disease. Nails may become brittle, hypertrophic and rough. Comparison of colour and trophic changes between limbs can give a good indication of the severity of peripheral arterial disease, unless there is bilateral disease, in which case the appearance of the limbs may approximate each other and examiner experience is required to judge severity (31,32).

Skin temperature and colour: skin colour is produced by blood in the subpapillary layer and varies with skin temperature, the position of the limb and the degree of oxygenation of the blood (reduced haemoglobin appears blue) (33).

Skin temperature is an indicator of the rate of blood flow in the dermal vessels, although the flow is governed primarily by constriction or dilatation of arterioles to maintain a constant core temperature. Skin temperature as a marker of perfusion is useful and can be assessed by lightly palpating the skin with the back of the hand and comparing similar sites from one limb to the other. An ischaemic limb is cold and temperature demarcation gives a rough indication of the level of occlusion. Assessment of temperature differences is confounded when both limbs are affected (30,32).

The Buerger test involves first elevating the foot with the patient supine and waiting until the veins have completely drained, and then placing the foot in a dependent position. Elevation of the limb above the level of central venous pressure (rarely more than 25 cm) allows pooled venous blood to drain, allowing an accurate assessment of the degree of arterial flow. The return time of blood to the dependent limb is a useful marker of disease severity (usually <20 seconds).(29,31)

- The normal limb will remain pink with elevation.
- Patients with significant peripheral arterial disease will have pallor of the feet with elevation and, in the declined position, there will be a dark flush extending proximally from the toes. The colour may be reddish or cyanotic depending on skin temperature (31).
- In patients with chronic arterial occlusion, arterioles are maximally dilated as a compensatory response to chronic ischaemia, which intensifies skin colour changes (31).
- It is important to differentiate blushing associated with arterial insufficiency from cellulitis accompanying an infectious process. A red, cellulitic appearance will persist despite elevation of the limb (30,31).
- In patients with acute arterial occlusion, the venules empty, resulting in a chalky white skin appearance regardless of the position of the extremities (31,32).

Ulceration: Ulcerations of the extremities have a characteristic appearance depending on their origin (table 6). Ulcerations caused by ischaemia are typically located at the termination of arterial branches. They are commonly found on the tips of the toes and between the toes. Ischaemic ulcers also form at sites of increased focal pressure, such as the lateral malleolus and metatarsal heads. The lesions often appear dry and punchy and are painful, but show little bleeding (Figure 2). Ischaemic ulcers are usually associated with other clinical features of chronic ischaemia, such as pallor, hair loss and nail changes, as mentioned above. (33,34)

*Table 6. **Foot ulcer differentiation***

Feature	Arterial ulcer	Venous ulcer	Neuropathic ulcer
Location	On toe joints, malleoli, anterior shin	Medial and lateral malleolar area above the bony prominence,	Plantar surface of the foot over the

	bone, base of the heel, pressure points	posterior part of the calf	metatarsal heads, heel, pressure points
Appearance	Irregular margins, dry and often pale or necrotic base	Irregular margins, pink or red base that may be covered with yellow fibrinous tissue	Punch ulcer, usually superficial but sometimes deep, with a red base
Ulcer within callus	Rare	No	Callous border, ulcer may be under a callus.
Foot temperature	Hot or cold	Hot	Hot
Pain	Yes, it can be severe	Yes, usually mild but can be severe.	No
Arterial pulses	Absent	Present	Absent or present
Sensation	Variable	Present	Absence of tactile, painful, thermal and vibratory sensations.
Foot deformities	No	No	Often
Skin changes	Shiny, tight hair, hair loss. Dependent blushing of leg and foot which pales with elevation of leg.	Erythema, bluish-brown pigmentation may be patchy or diffuse: "stasis" changes; white atrophy, oedema; dry skin; varicose veins common.	Waxy or shiny, hair loss, may be tight; skin dry; may have non-pitting oedema, especially on dorsum of foot.
Reflections	Present	Present	Absent

Some patients have combined arterial and venous disease and manifest signs of both arterial and venous insufficiency, including ulcers of mixed aetiology. Similarly, patients with diabetes may have arterial disease and peripheral neuropathy, each of which may contribute to ulcer formation. (32,34)

Figure 2. Ulcer on external aspect of distal leg region (From: McGee, 1998).

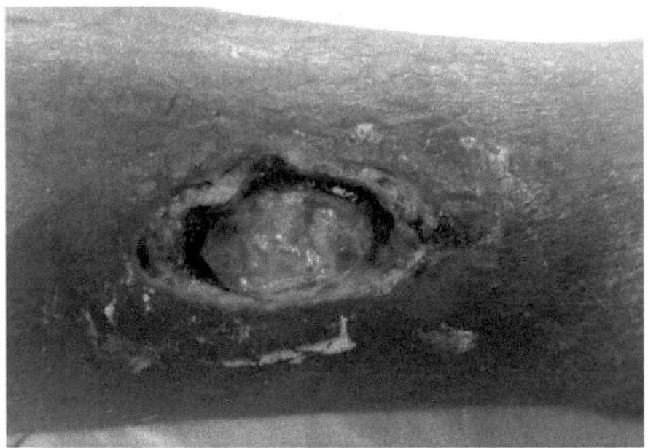

Gangrene: In addition to ulcers, patients may have frankly gangrenous toes, either in the forefoot or hindfoot. Gangrene can be described as dry or wet. Dry gangrene is characterised by a hard, dry texture, usually appearing on the distal part of the fingers and toes, often with a clear demarcation between viable and black necrotic tissue. This form of gangrene is common in patients with peripheral arterial disease. Wet gangrene is characterised by a wet appearance, extensive swelling and blistering. Wet gangrene represents a surgical emergency and appropriate consultation should be made when it is identified (30,33).

Pulses: Assessment of pulses in the patient with suspected peripheral arterial disease should include palpation of the brachial, radial, femoral, popliteal, dorsalis pedis and posterior tibial arteries. The normal popliteal artery is often not easily palpated, but can usually be identified with Doppler. Evaluation of murmurs with a stethoscope over the iliac arteries should also be performed. Inability to easily palpate a particular vessel should lead to interrogation with hand-held continuous wave Doppler ultrasound (31,32).

Bedside ankle-arm index: The resting ankle-brachial systolic pressure index is a simple test that can be performed at the bedside and should be measured in patients with one or more findings consistent with peripheral arterial disease on review of symptoms or other findings on physical examination. The ankle brachial index is the ratio of the ankle systolic blood pressure divided by the brachial systolic pressure detected with a Doppler probe. In patients without symptoms or with mild to moderate symptoms, an ankle-arm index of <0.90 has a high degree of sensitivity and specificity for peripheral arterial disease, using arteriography as a reference standard.(33,34)

An attempt can be made to obtain an ankle-arm index in patients with more severe ischaemia at the bedside; however, the patient may not tolerate inflation of the blood pressure cuff on the affected limb, and Doppler signals in the foot vessels may be too weak to accurately measure shear pressures (32).

Calculation of the ankle-arm index is a relatively simple and inexpensive method to confirm clinical suspicion of lower extremity arterial stenosis or occlusion. The highest resting systolic blood pressure at the ankle is compared to the highest systolic brachial pressure, and the ratio of the two pressures defines the ankle-arm index. For patients with peripheral arterial disease, the ankle-arm index provides a measure of disease severity and predicts coronary and cerebrovascular disease. (31,32)

Neurological assessment: Neurological examination of the lower extremities is important and should include motor and sensory testing. In the patient with acute limb ischaemia, sensory loss and progressive motor loss of the lower extremities are ominous signs indicating the need for immediate intervention. Patients with acute arterial or graft thrombosis superimposed on chronic ischaemia may be more tolerant depending on the efficacy of the collateral vessels. (32,33)

Chronic ischaemia can cause various patterns of sensory loss, progressing from distal to proximal as the severity of ischaemia worsens. Diabetic patients may have an overlapping sensory neuropathy, which typically has a glove-and-a-half distribution and reduces the sense of vibration and two-point discrimination. The use of monofilament calipers (Semmel-Weinstein) is a good objective way to assess diabetic neuropathy (31,34).

<u>**Diagnosis**</u>

For the diagnosis of PAD, an adequate clinical history with the presence of a history of risk factors or symptoms of peripheral arterial disease, together with the findings of an adequate physical examination (previously described), is sufficient to establish the diagnosis of peripheral arterial disease (32).

When patients presenting with typical symptoms of arterial obstruction present symptoms of intermittent claudication, this represents the tip of the iceberg of a major epidemiological problem, as they tend to think that these symptoms are due to problems related to their age. On the other hand, there are patients with atypical symptoms or with dubious pulse examination, for which the ankle-arm index (with or without exercise) is diagnostic of arterial obstruction if it is ≤0.9 . (30,31)

Abnormal arterial examination/tissue loss: In patients with risk factors for PAD and no history of symptoms suggestive of an alternative vascular process (e.g., abdominal or back pain as in aortic dissection), the presence of obvious abnormalities on pulse examination, ischaemia, pain at rest or tissue loss strongly suggests the presence of PAD. (29,32)

Abnormal ankle-brachial index: Although history, symptoms, physical examination and bedside ABI may strongly suggest a diagnosis of PAD, they are often not specific or sensitive enough to judge the severity of the disease or to pinpoint sites of obstruction. Depending on the clinical presentation, formal ABI testing or additional studies may be indicated. These may include other physiological tests in a vascular laboratory (treadmill exercise test, segmental pressures or pulse volume recordings) or vascular imaging (figure 3) (27,34).

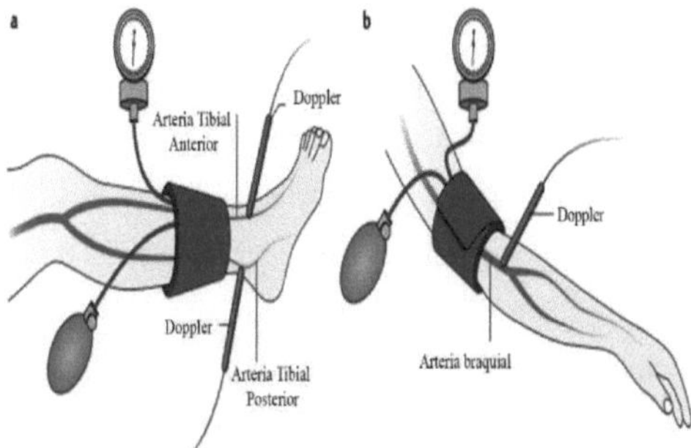

Figure 3. Measurement and calculation of the ankle-brachial index (ABI) in the diagnosis of peripheral arterial disease. ABI is the ratio of a| the highest systolic blood pressure between the posterior tibial artery and the dorsal artery of the foot to b| the highest systolic blood pressure between the two arms (16).

For patients with risk factors for peripheral arterial disease and symptoms of leg strain (claudication, atypical pain), formal vascular laboratory tests are suggested to confirm the diagnosis (35).

The need for testing in patients with tissue loss should be individualised. For most patients, formal vascular laboratory studies are suggested, whenever possible, prior to vascular intervention (35,37).

An abnormal ankle-brachial index (≤0.9) has excellent overall accuracy for detecting arterial stenosis ≥50 per cent using arteriography as standard. For most patients with exertional limb pain (classic claudication, atypical symptoms), an ABI ≤0.9 is diagnostic of peripheral arterial disease, particularly in the context of adequate clinical history. However, other non-atherosclerotic pathological processes may also cause arterial occlusion and an abnormal ABI (e.g., thrombosed popliteal aneurysm), and need to be distinguished from atherosclerosis (36).

There is a general, but not absolute, correlation between symptoms and the site and severity of peripheral arterial disease, and severity is estimated from the ankle-brachial index:

- An ankle brachial index >0.9 with an upper limit of 1.3 generally excludes clinically significant arterial occlusive disease. Typically, the pressure is higher in the ankle than in the arm (i.e. ankle-arm index >1 to 1.3). An ankle brachial index of 0.9 to 0.99 is classified as borderline normal (28,31).

- An ankle-arm index >1.3 suggests the presence of non-compressible calcified vessels and the need for additional vascular studies, such as pulse volume recordings, measurement of toe and index toe-arm pressures, transcutaneous oxygen measurements or arterial duplex studies (28,31).

- An ankle-arm index ≤0.9 is diagnostic of occlusive arterial disease in patients with symptoms of claudication or other signs of ischaemia and has a sensitivity of 95 % (and specificity of 100 %) for detecting occlusive lesions with positive arteriogram associated with ≥50 % stenosis in one or more large vessels.(28,31)

- An ankle-arm index of 0.4 to 0.9 suggests a degree of arterial obstruction often associated with claudication (28,31).

- An ankle brachial index below 0.4 generally represents multilevel disease (any combination of iliac, femoral or tibial vessel disease) and may be associated with non-healing ulcerations, ischaemic pain at rest or gangrene of the foot (28,31).

These positive physical examination findings then help physicians diagnose the presence of peripheral arterial disease: abnormal pedal pulse, unilaterally cold extremity, prolonged venous filling time, and a femoral murmur. Other physical signs help determine the extent and distribution of vascular disease, including an abnormal femoral pulse, lower extremity murmurs, warm knees and Buerger's test. Capillary refill test and findings of discolouration of the feet, atrophic skin and hairless extremities do not help in diagnostic decisions (28,29).

Questionnaires

A number of questionnaires have been used to detect the presence of intermittent claudication in a standardised way. Currently, the San Diego Claudication Questionnaire (SDCQ)12 and the Edinburgh Claudication Questionnaire (ECQ)13 show sensitivity, and all have excellent specificity. These questionnaires have been translated into other languages, but further validated translations are required to enable their use worldwide. (29,32)

Although the use of these questionnaires, in addition to measurement of the ankle-arm index, provides more accurate data on the prevalence of symptomatic and asymptomatic peripheral arterial disease, these questionnaires have limitations in that they do not cover the full range of symptomatic disease. In fact, many patients may have an atypical presentation of claudication, or have no pain because they do not walk enough due to other comorbidities (29,32).

Site and severity of peripheral arterial disease

Segmental pressure and pulse volume recordings: Segmental pressure and pulse volume recordings, which are physiological studies performed in the vascular laboratory, are useful in confirming a diagnosis of suspected peripheral arterial disease in the lower extremities based on clinical history and physical examination, and in determining the site and severity of the disease. (33)

These studies include formal ankle-brachial index tests and are performed on both legs. Measurement of toe/toe-arm pressure is an alternative to the ankle-arm index for establishing a diagnosis of PAD in patients with non-compressible vessels (usually patients with long-standing or elderly diabetes) (31,33).

Stress testing: Some patients with peripheral arterial disease who have a classic history of claudication and others with atypical limb pain have a normal resting ankle-arm index (0.91 to 1.30). For these patients, stress testing is indicated. Abnormal exercise ankle-arm indexes support a diagnosis of peripheral arterial disease as the aetiology of their symptoms. Treadmill exercise testing is useful in providing the most objective evidence of the magnitude of functional limitation in patients with claudication and can also be used to guide response to treatment (30,32).

Vascular imaging:

Vascular imaging is generally not necessary to establish a diagnosis of peripheral arterial disease; however, it may be indicated to differentiate peripheral arterial disease from other vascular aetiologies as a source of arterial obstruction, if peripheral arterial disease is questioned as the primary aetiology of symptoms (e.g., arterial aneurysm or thromboembolism is suspected). However, vascular imaging is necessary to identify appropriate targets for intervention and for continued surveillance after intervention. Contrast arteriography (figure 4) remains the gold standard for evaluation of the threatened limb. A complete bilateral study of the aortic, iliac, femoral, popliteal and run-off vessels should be performed in patients in whom revascularisation is expected, provided that there are no contraindications.(33,34)

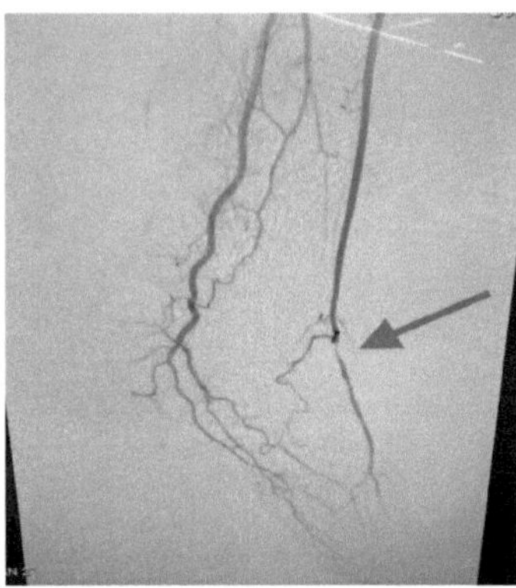

However, vascular imaging is necessary to identify appropriate targets for intervention and for ongoing post-intervention surveillance (34,35).

Laboratory studies: There is no specific biomarker for peripheral arterial disease. Routine laboratory studies include complete blood count with differential, metabolic panel, lipid profile, and possibly homocysteine, lipoprotein A and C-reactive protein. (32,34)

A diagnostic algorithm for peripheral arterial disease is presented below (Figure 5).

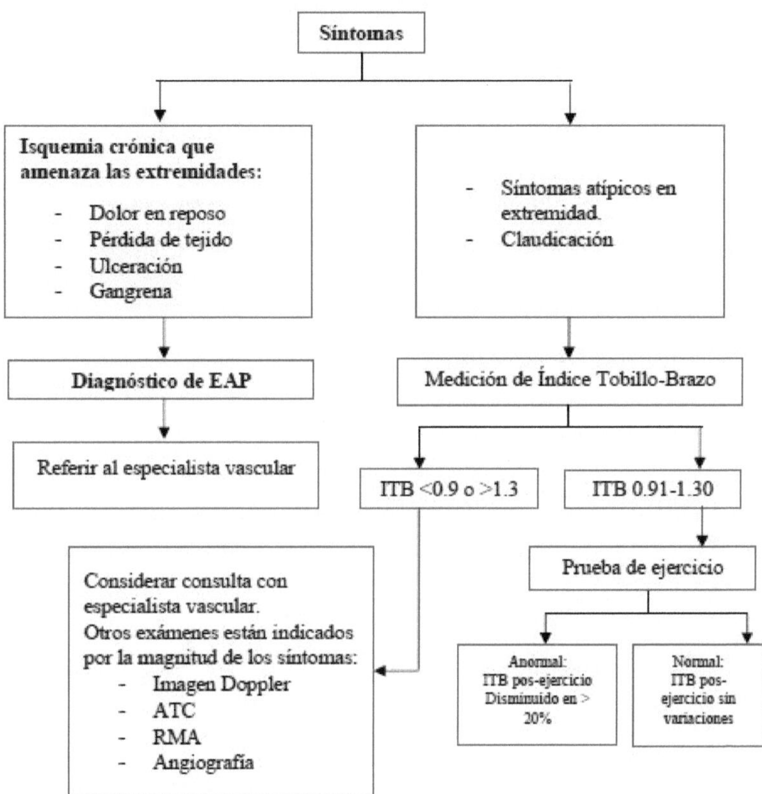

ATC: Angiografía tomográfica computarizada, RMA: Angiografía por resonancia magnética, ITB: Índice tobillo brazo, EAP: Enfermedad arterial periférica.

<u>**Differential Diagnosis**</u>

Other causes of arterial obstruction: Any vascular disease resulting in arterial stenosis or occlusion can cause symptoms of limb pain or tissue loss. These include arterial thrombosis due to aneurysm, arterial injury, arterial dissection or thromboembolism, among others. Arterial imaging of the lower extremities differentiates many of these aetiologies from each other. (32,35)

- **Arterial aneurysm:** The popliteal artery is the most common site of a peripheral arterial aneurysm causing symptoms of lower limb ischaemia, which is due to thrombosis of the aneurysm. The presence of a peripheral aneurysm should prompt evaluation for other aneurysms. (31,33)

- **Arterial dissection:** Arterial dissection can cause ischaemia in the lower extremities; however, acute dissection is usually accompanied by sudden focal pain overlying the affected artery. For aortic dissection, pain often begins in the chest and moves to the abdomen or pelvis as the dissection progresses. After instrumentation, focal areas of dissection may appear in the region of the arterial access. A history of previous pain or a previous interventional procedure distinguishes them from PAD; however, peripheral arterial disease may overlap. (32,35)

- **Embolism:** debris from proximal sources may embolise distal to the toes or more proximally, causing acute limb ischaemia. The more acute time course of symptoms generally distinguishes these patients from patients with PAD. (33,34)

- **Popliteal impingement syndrome:** Popliteal impingement syndrome may also present with intermittent claudication and should be suspected in the young patient who presents with claudication but lacks atherosclerotic risk factors. Popliteal entrapment syndrome, which is due to abnormal musculoskeletal insertions or an abnormal course of the popliteal artery, leads to compression of the popliteal artery with activity (32,34).

- **Cystic disease of the adventitia:** Cystic disease of the adventitia is a rare entity that can lead to arterial obstruction related to mucoid degeneration of the artery. When it occurs in the femoral or popliteal artery, claudication symptoms are indistinguishable from popliteal atherosclerotic disease. Patients tend to be younger and typical risk factors for cardiovascular disease are often absent (31,34).

- **Thromboangiitis obliterans (Buerger's disease):** Thromboangiitis obliterans, also called Buerger's disease, is an inflammatory, segmental, non-atherosclerotic disease that most commonly affects the small to medium-sized arteries and veins of the extremities. Patients are younger than typical patients with atherosclerotic vascular disease and are heavy smokers. Ischaemia of the fingers is the most common presentation and, although involvement of larger arteries is uncommon, claudication may occur, but is almost always associated with signs of distal ischaemia. (32,34)

- **Other vascular disorders:** other vascular aetiologies that can cause lower limb ischaemia include trauma to the limbs, radiation arteritis, vasculitis or ergot use for migraines. In endurance athletes, especially cyclists, an even more unusual cause of claudication is due to repeated trauma (stretching or twisting) of the external iliac artery, which can lead to endofibrosis of the vessel. (33,35)

Non-arterial aetiologies of limb pain: The aetiology of limb pain can be divided into categories including vascular (arterial or venous), neurogenic and musculoskeletal causes. Arterial causes were previously discussed in the previous section. Non-arterial pathological conditions should also be considered in the differential diagnosis of limb pain. The main clinical features that distinguish these disorders from arterial claudication are (31,32):

- Neurological pain is predominantly due to neurospinal (e.g. disc disease, spinal stenosis, tumour) or neuropathic (e.g. diabetes, alcohol abuse) causes. Neurogenic claudication, also called "spinal claudication" or "pseudoclaudication", describes a pain syndrome due to compression of the lumbar neurospinal canal, which is usually due to osteophytic narrowing of the neurospinal canal. (31,32) The clinical presentation often helps to distinguish vasculogenic (i.e. true) claudication from pseudoclaudication. Unlike true claudication, which occurs with walking and is relieved by standing, pseudoclaudication causes pain with upright posture (lumbar lordosis) and is relieved by sitting or lying down. Symptoms in patients with pseudoclaudication may also be relieved by leaning forward and straightening the spine (usually done by pushing a shopping trolley or leaning against a wall). (31,33)
- Musculoskeletal pain is derived from the bones, joints, ligaments, tendons and fascial elements of the lower extremity (32).
- Osteoarthritis of the hip or knee joints can be distinguished clinically from aortoiliac disease because the pain of osteoarthritis may not disappear quickly after exercise, may be associated with climatic changes, and may vary in intensity from day to day (usually worse

in the morning or on waking). A similar distinction applies to foot and ankle arthritis that produces pain not attributable to peripheral arterial disease. (32,34)

- Baker's cysts can also cause lower extremity pain that does not follow the pattern of peripheral artery disease claudication pain on exertion that resolves rapidly with rest. (31,35)

- Nocturnal leg cramps occur among elderly and ill patients and, unlike claudication, are not associated with exercise. This complaint is thought to be neuromuscular rather than vascular in origin (31,35).

- Calf pressure and stiffness is a complaint mainly seen in athletes and is usually associated with chronic exercise. It is thought to be due to increased compartment pressure and may persist even after rest (31,35).

- Chronic venous disease can cause "venous claudication", but is usually easily distinguished from arterial claudication by a varying degree of limb swelling or varicosities and greater discomfort with limb dependence. (31,35)

Several of the entities considered within the differential diagnosis can be found in table 7.

Table 7. Differential diagnosis of Peripheral Artery Disease (12)

Potential aetiology	Diagnostic Tracks
Musculoskeletal Arthritis (hip, knee, ankle) Chronic compartment syndrome Medial tibial stress syndrome Muscle contracture	Painful discomfort, often with exertion or weight-bearing activities Tight calf pain that occurs after intense exercise in athletes with large muscle mass; relieves slowly with rest. Anterior pain that improves with rest; possible localised tenderness. History of trauma or overuse; possible ecchymosis; pain caused by use of the affected muscle group.
Neurological Nerve entrapment nerve root compression (e.g. herniated disc, radiculopathy) Peripheral neuropathy (diabetes mellitus, alcohol abuse). Spinal stenosis	Tingling and numbness in the affected nerve distribution; may progress to muscle weakness and atrophy. Posterior radiating pain originating in the back, often changes with position and improves with lumbar extension; possible weakness or motor or sensory changes Distal pain, tingling, numbness or weakness that may follow a sock-like distribution. Low back pain radiating to bilateral lower extremities with numbness, weakness and fatigue.

Vascular	
Deep vein thrombosis	May be unilateral; often associated with swelling or tenderness; history of immobility or other risk factors.
Popliteal arterial entrapment	Pain on exertion; more common in men; common in young, active patients.
Vasculitis	Possible skin findings or other systemic symptoms; family or personal history of inflammatory or autoimmune disorders.
Venous insufficiency	Probable swelling; symptoms may progress proximally

<u>**Management**</u>

The management of patients with PAD of the lower limbs is aimed at relieving symptoms and reducing the risk of progression of cardiovascular disease and its complications (37).

Management of PAD includes smoking cessation, exercise, a strict dietary regimen, and in addition pharmacological treatment with statins to achieve a target low-density lipoprotein level of 100 mg/dL or less, and antiplatelet therapy with 75 to 325 mg aspirin or 75 mg clopidogrel daily. Patients with lifestyle-limiting claudication should be considered for a trial of cilostazol in the absence of heart failure. (47)

1. Lifestyle modification

Smoking cessation

Smoking is closely related to the development of atherosclerosis either directly or indirectly, in fact, it corresponds to the most important risk factor for the development of claudication. Total and permanent smoking cessation represents the most clinically cost-effective intervention in patients with atherosclerosis. Simple advice is often not very effective, as smoking is a form of addiction (37,38).

The combination of exercise therapy and smoking cessation may also be beneficial. Finally, adjunctive treatments such as nicotine replacement therapy and bupropion (an inhibitor of the neuronal uptake of norepinephrine, serotonin and dopamine) have been successful in increasing the likelihood of permanent smoking cessation. (38)

Exercise

The risk of peripheral arterial disease is inversely related to previous levels of physical activity and is therefore a protective factor. Walking ability has been shown to increase with physical training in patients with claudication and regular exercise together with risk factor modification, especially smoking cessation, is the cornerstone of conservative therapy for intermittent claudication. (37,39)

Exercise in peripheral arterial disease generally consists of treadmill walking, although other modalities, such as upper limb exercise and barbell strides, have been reported (38,19).

In addition, exercise-induced improvement in walking ability results in improvement in routine daily activities and exercise rehabilitation itself is associated with minimal morbidity and mortality (38).

Diet and weight loss

There is evidence that patients with atherosclerotic disease should follow a low-fat diet, as well as evidence for the benefit of a Mediterranean-style diet.(39)

In addition, weight control has been proposed to be an essential feature of the overall management strategy for peripheral arterial disease since obesity is associated with increased relative risks of total mortality and cardiovascular disease. Abdominal fat distribution, but not total body fat, is associated with peripheral arterial occlusive disease, independent of concurrent cardiovascular risk factors. (38,40)

On this basis, every overweight patient with peripheral arterial disease should be given an optimal dietary plan and a weight loss goal (41).

Fibre intake is also suggested as it interferes with the micellar absorption of dietary cholesterol. Increased fibre intake is associated with a lower incidence of peripheral arterial disease. However, to date, there is no evidence that a diet rich in fruits and vegetables protects against peripheral arterial disease, although a modest benefit cannot be excluded. (38,41)

With regard to sodium restriction, sodium restriction has been recommended for hypertensives. Patients with peripheral arterial disease develop a greater degree of cardiac hypertrophy than other hypertensive patients with the same level of mean arterial pressure. Furthermore, being an atherosclerotic disease, it is closely related to the development of hypertension and sodium restriction is recommended in these patients. (38,40)

Finally, with regard to fish oil consumption, although there are some beneficial effects on haemodynamic parameters, there is no evidence of improved clinical outcomes (40).

Diabetes

Given that intermittent claudication is about twice as common among diabetic patients as among non-diabetic patients and that the association between diabetes mellitus and the development of peripheral arterial disease has been established and is more aggressive in patients with diabetes, therefore, strict dietary control is necessary to achieve adequate glycaemic control in order to limit vascular damage to the extremities. (40)

The UK Prospective Diabetes Study (UKPDS) has demonstrated a significant reduction in any diabetes endpoint (mainly microvascular) after tight glycaemic control. These data seem robust enough to make good diabetes control a priority in patients with peripheral arterial disease. (39,41)

Alcohol

An inverse association between alcohol consumption and peripheral arterial disease has been reported in the non-smoking population. On the other hand, with increased consumption there is an increased risk of hypertension and other cardiac and non-cardiac diseases resulting in increased morbidity and premature mortality. The data are probably not strong enough to emphasise alcohol consumption as part of the lifestyle approach to peripheral arterial disease. (39,49)

Antioxidants

Decreased levels of antioxidants are closely related to the development of peripheral arterial disease, especially vitamin E and C have been implicated. The Rotterdam study reported a significant inverse effect of vitamin C intake on the prevalence of PAD in women and a similar effect of vitamin E in men; despite this, evidence has shown no benefit from vitamin E supplementation. Thus, a Cochrane review of five studies concluded that there was insufficient evidence to recommend its use in claudication at present (41).

2. Medical treatment

Lipid-lowering treatments in PAD

Based on the knowledge that elevated lipid levels are associated with increased cardiovascular risk in patients with peripheral arterial disease; the 2019 European Society of Cardiology dyslipidaemia guidelines recommend C-LDL targets according to the 10-

year risk of fatal cardiovascular events. Patients with PAD belong to the very high-risk category, with ≥10% risk of a fatal cardiovascular event. In these patients, both LDL-C reduction by≥50% from baseline and an LDL-C goal of<55 mg/dL (<1.4 mmol/L) are recommended. (41,42)

To achieve this LDL-C target, treatment with a high-intensity statin at the maximum tolerated dose is recommended as this is supported by definitive evidence of benefit on cardiovascular morbidity and mortality; in addition there is also support for positive effects of lipid lowering on major adverse limb events as well as on gait performance in patients with peripheral arterial disease. If patients cannot reach the target or report intolerance to statins, a combination of statins (at a lower dose if statin intolerant) with ezetimibe and additionally with the addition of a PCSK9 inhibitor is recommended (41).

Antithrombotic therapies in peripheral arterial disease

Current treatment of symptomatic peripheral arterial disease comprises antiplatelet monotherapy (either aspirin 75-100 mg per day or clopidogrel 75 mg per day), with improved benefit from more intense antiplatelet therapy (42).

Dual antiplatelet therapy should be given for at least one month after drug-coated balloon angioplasty, and for 3 months after drug release or covered stent (42,43). (42,43)

Finally, based on the results of the VOYAGER study, combination therapy with aspirin (100 mg/day) and rivaroxaban (2 x 2.5 mg/day) should be considered for dual therapy post-intervention. (42)

Anticoagulation

Warfarin

Although there are studies supporting the use of warfarin with aspirin for the prevention of complications in patients with a history of acute coronary syndrome, for patients with peripheral arterial disease they did not show promising results. The WAVE trial investigated the use of warfarin anticoagulation in combination with aspirin for patients with symptomatic peripheral arterial disease (81.8% of the total trial population), subclavian disease and carotid disease. The trial found no significant difference in the occurrence of major adverse cardiovascular events among patients receiving combined therapy of aspirin and warfarin alone; on the other hand, an increased risk of intracranial bleeding was found in these patients. (42,44)

In view of the above, Warfarin is not indicated for use in patients with peripheral arterial disease.

Rivaroxaban

The COMPASS study demonstrated improved mortality with low-dose rivaroxaban (2.5 mg twice daily) in combination with aspirin for patients with peripheral artery disease. Although bleeding events are more frequent with the use of aspirin with rivaroxaban or rivaroxaban alone, neither regimen was associated with fatal or intracranial bleeding. (43)

Peripheral vasodilators

Intermittent claudication results from peripheral ischaemia distal to a stenosis under stress. This mismatch between tissue supply and demand is often the result of stenosis, whereby an insufficient vasodilator response may result in symptoms that are relieved by rest. As such, peripheral vasodilators are potentially beneficial for claudication, which is why the ACC/AHA guidelines include a class IA recommendation for cilostazol in the treatment of symptomatic claudication. (42,44)

Multiple trials have evaluated its usefulness in symptomatic claudication, finding that cilostazol increases exercise tolerance compared to placebo at a dose of 100 mg twice daily. Common adverse events include headache, palpitations and diarrhoea, and cilostazol is contraindicated in patients with heart failure, as drugs in this class may be associated with excess mortality. (41,44)

The side effect profile, contraindication for heart failure, the number of pills patients often take (diabetes, hypertension, etc.) and the subtle benefit are reasons why cilostazol is used infrequently and should only be considered in medically optimised patients with refractory claudication who can tolerate the drug. (42,43)

3. Treatment based on revascularisation. -

Without revascularisation, peripheral arterial disease of a limb often results in the loss of the limb. However, neither open surgical revascularisation nor endovascular treatment (EVT) guarantees treatment success and freedom from restenosis and revascularisation failure. Today, managing the risk of revascularisation failure is one of the major challenges in the vascular field. (42,43)

The goals of VTE in patients affected by peripheral arterial disease are pain relief, wound healing and functional preservation of limbs. However, revascularisation can cause morbidity, which correlates with many hospital admissions, ongoing outpatient care and significant treatment and medical care costs, as well as mortality. Therefore, it is necessary to identify patients for whom VTE may be beneficial to avoid potential failure. (41,43)

Patient risk estimation

Peripheral arterial disease generally affects patients with advanced age and multiple comorbidities. In this context, estimation of operative risk and life expectancy is critical. Preoperative anaesthetic and cardiac assessment prior to limb revascularisation is mandatory. Several procedural risk factors have been identified for the peripheral arterial disease population, these are: advanced age (over 75 years), coronary artery disease, congestive heart failure, diabetes mellitus (DM), chronic kidney disease (CKD), smoking, cerebrovascular disease, elevated body mass index, dementia, functional status and frailty. (42,43)

4. Follow-up

After initial counselling, a three-month follow-up should be scheduled to assess risk reduction strategies and the effectiveness of exercise therapy and medical therapies to reduce symptoms. (42)

Patients who show improvement and who are satisfied with their progress can be scheduled for an annual vascular examination, which should include an ankle-brachial index test. In the meantime, it is not necessary to repeat non-invasive vascular studies unless there is a significant change in symptoms (41,43).

Non-compliance, in particular continued smoking, remains a major problem in the treatment of patients with peripheral arterial disease. Those who continue to smoke should again be warned about the increased risk of progression of peripheral arterial disease. Most vascular physicians are generally reluctant to suggest intervention (open or percutaneous) in patients with claudication who continue to smoke because of poorer overall outcomes. (42,43)

Management of chronic limb-threatening ischaemia

For the management of chronic limb-threatening ischaemia, initial medical treatment of chronic limb-threatening ischaemia includes appropriate analgesia and intravenous administration of unfractionated heparin (UFH): initially 5 000 IU, or 70-100 IU/kg, followed by infusion, dose adjusted to patient response and monitored by activated clotting time or activated partial thromboplastin time (aPTT) (44,45).

The aim is to further reduce embolism or clot propagation and provide an anti-inflammatory effect. Although this approach is widely accepted, no recent randomised study has been conducted to confirm the benefit of UFH for ICAE, nor has any randomised study compared unfractionated UFH with other anticoagulants. A primary outcome in chronic limb-threatening ischaemia is to extend amputation-free survival. Major amputation (above the ankle) in ICAE is necessary and indicated in the presence of life-threatening infection, when pain cannot be controlled at rest, or when extensive necrosis has occurred that has destroyed the foot. (44,45)

Revascularisation therapy can be either surgical or endovascular. Both surgical bypass and percutaneous transluminal angioplasty (PTA) are potential approaches for revascularisation of peripheral arterial disease. However, these approaches do not provide the same results. While the scheme developed by the TransAtlantic Intersociety Consensus II is widely used whereby each lesion can be approached from an anatomical perspective (Table 8), the GLASS scale allows for more specific decision making (Table 9). (45,46)

Table 8. Approach scheme according to TransAtlantic Intersociety Consensus II

Type	Approach
A	Lesions that give excellent results and should be treated by endovascular means
B	They offer sufficiently good results with endovascular methods that this approach is the preferred first choice, unless open revascularisation is required for other associated lesions.
C	They produce superior long-term results with open revascularisation, and endovascular methods should be used only in patients at high risk of open repair.
D	Most suitable for surgical revascularisation and when an endovascular approach is not warranted.

Without revascularisation, up to 40% of patients with ICAE will require lower limb amputation within 1 year.

Table 9. **(A) Original/composite femoropopliteal (FP) disease classification in GLASS. (B) Original/composite infrapopliteal (IP) disease classification in GLASS.**

	A. Femoro-Popliteal (FP) classification
0	Mild or non-significant disease (<50%)
1	Total length AFS disease <1/3 (<10 cm); may include a single focal CTO (<5 cm) provided there is no flush occlusion; popliteal artery with mild or no significant disease.
2	Total length of AFS disease 1/3-2/3 (10-20 cm); may include CTO with a total of <1/3 (10 cm) but not flush occlusion; Focal stenosis of popliteal artery <2 cm, without trifurcation involvement.
3	Total length AFS disease >2/3 (>20 cm) in length; may include any flush occlusion <20 cm or non-flush CTO 10 to 20 cm in length; Short popliteal stenosis 2 to 5 cm, without trifurcation involvement.
4	AFS occlusion of total length >20 cm; popliteal disease > 5 cm or extending to the trifurcation; any popliteal CTO.
	B. Infra-Plopitea (IP) classification
0	Mild or non-significant disease (<50%)
1	Focal stenosis < 3 cm excluding tibioperoneal trunk
2	Total length of target artery disease <1/3 (<10 cm); single focal CTO (<3 cm not including tibioperoneal trunk and origin of target artery)
3	Total length of target artery disease 1/3-2/3 (10-20 cm); CTO 3-10 cm (may include the origin of the target artery, but not the tibioperoneal trunk)
4	Total length of target artery disease > 2/3 length; CTO >1/3 (>10 cm) length (may include the origin of the target artery); any CTO of the tibioperoneal trunk

SFA: Superficial Femoral Artery, CTO: Chronic Total Obstruction

Percutaneous transluminal angioplasty, also called balloon angioplasty, for the treatment of occlusive arterial disease relies on several mechanisms to increase the diameter of the arterial lumen. The deployment of a stent during this process helps to increase the lumen area by providing a scaffold for the artery wall that almost completely prevents elastic recoil. Endovascular therapy has also evolved with improved techniques and technologies (45,47).

It is important to note that many of the devices were approved for use in patients with claudication, and not ICAE, due to trial design to limit patients with worse outcomes. Despite this limitation, current data suggest that bare metal stents have an advantage over balloon angioplasty in intermediate and long superficial femoral artery lesions, and self-expanding drug-eluting stents have demonstrated superior patency at 2 years over balloon angioplasty with provisional stenting.(45,48)

In surgical revascularisation, accurate preoperative planning is essential. The autogenous ipsilateral saphenous vein is the preferred conduit for infrainguinal bypass grafts. A high-quality conduit is critical for a successful bypass and has direct implications for short- and long-term patency outcomes (46).

On the other hand, pharmacological normalisation of microcirculatory changes may improve the results of revascularisation and is the only option in patients in whom revascularisation is impossible or has failed. Prostanoids act by preventing platelet and leukocyte activation and protect the vascular endothelium. A recent systematic review and meta-analysis on the use of prostanoids for ICAE included 20 RCTs with a total of 2724 participants. Compared to placebo, prostanoids show significantly greater efficacy in the treatment of pain at rest (RR: 1.32, 95% CI: 1.10-1.57) and ulcer healing (RR: 1.54, 95% CI: 1.22-1.96). There was no statistically significant effect on the number of amputations and mortality when prostanoids were examined as a drug class, but iloprost showed favourable results in reducing major amputations (above/below knee) (RR 0.69, 95% CI 0.52-0.93). (45,47)

Cilostazol is a phosphodiesterase inhibitor that acts on cyclic adenosine monophosphate. It is a direct arterial vasodilator and also inhibits platelet aggregation. Cilostazol is used to treat the symptoms of intermittent claudication, but its use for chronic limb-threatening ischaemia is less well studied, so there is no strong evidence that cilostazol improves clinical outcomes in patients with chronic limb-threatening ischaemia. (46,47)

Finally, other therapeutic approaches, such as spinal cord stimulation, hyperbaric therapy and regenerative therapies, including gene therapy, stem cell therapies, have been tried in patients with peripheral arterial disease and chronic ischaemia threatening the non-revascularisable limb, with inconclusive results. (48,49)

CONCLUSIONS

Peripheral arterial disease is a disease caused by a decrease in arterial blood flow secondary to atherosclerosis, leading to impaired peripheral circulation. It is much more common in developing countries. The risk factors for the development of peripheral arterial disease are the same as for any other cardiovascular disease, including non-modifiable risk factors (age, female sex and black race) and modifiable risk factors (diabetes mellitus, dyslipidaemia, hypertension, hyperhomocysteinemia).

It may be asymptomatic, but as the narrowing of the vascular lumen progresses, clinical manifestations (intermittent claudication, pain at rest, ulceration and gangrene) occur. To classify the clinical stage of the patient, one of the tools used is the Fontaine Clinical Classification.

For the diagnosis of peripheral arterial disease, an adequate clinical history is required (history of risk factors or compatible symptoms), in addition to an adequate physical examination showing a decrease/absence of the amplitude of the distal pulses as well as trophic changes in the affected limb. On the other hand, there are patients with atypical symptoms or with a dubious pulse examination, for which the ankle-arm index (with or without exercise) is used, and a diagnosis of arterial obstruction is made if it is ≤ 0.9.

Treatment of peripheral arterial disease involves lifestyle changes (physical exercise, diet and weight loss, smoking cessation) in addition to pharmacological treatment (statins, antiplatelet therapy) and in cases where there is a significant impact on quality of life, a trial of cilostazol may be considered in the absence of heart failure.

Surgical treatment (open surgical revascularisation or endovascular treatment) does not guarantee successful treatment and freedom from restenosis and revascularisation failure. Currently, managing the risk of revascularisation failure is one of the major challenges in the vascular field.

BIBLIOGRAPHY

1. Aboyans V, Ricco JB, Bartelink ML, Björck M, Brodmann M, & et al. (2018). Editor's Choice e 2017 ESC Guidelines on the Diagnosis and Treatment of Peripheral Arterial Diseases, in collaboration with the European Society for Vascular Surgery (ESVS). Eur J Vasc Endovasc Surg (2018).

2. Bolaños I, Chaves A, Gallón L, Ibañez M, & López H. (2018). Peripheral arterial disease in lower limbs. Revista Medicina Legal de Costa Rica.

3. Brunton S, Anderson J, & Vacalis S. (2021). Updates in the Management of Peripheral Arterial Disease: Focus on Reduction of Atherothrombotic Risk. Supplement to The Journal of Family Practice | Vol 70, No 8.

4. Conte S, & Vale P. (2017). Peripheral Arterial Disease. Heart, Lung and Circulation, Volume 27, Issue 4, P427-432.

5. Hamburg NM, Creager MA. Pathophysiology of Intermittent Claudication in Peripheral Artery Disease. Circ J. 2017 Feb 24;81(3):281-289. doi: 10.1253/circj.CJ-16-1286. Epub 2017 Jan 26. PMID: 28123169.

6. Criqui M, & Aboyans V. (2015). Epidemiology of Peripheral Artery Disease. Circulation Research Compendium on Peripheral Artery Disease/AHA.116.303849.

7. Fowkes FG, Rudan D, Rudan I, et al. Comparison of global estimates of prevalence and risk factors for peripheral artery disease in 2000 and 2010: a systematic review and analysis. Lancet 2013; 382:1329.

8. Eraso LH, Fukaya E, Mohler ER 3rd, et al. Peripheral arterial disease, prevalence and cumulative risk factor profile analysis. Eur J Prev Cardiol 2014; 21:704.

9. Kröger K, Stang A, Kondratieva J, et al. Prevalence of peripheral arterial disease - results of the Heinz Nixdorf recall study. Eur J Epidemiol 2006; 21:279.

10. Kullo IJ, Bailey KR, Kardia SL, et al. Ethnic differences in peripheral arterial disease in the NHLBI Genetic Epidemiology Network of Arteriopathy (GENOA) study. Vasc Med 2003; 8:237.

11. Leeper NJ, Kullo IJ, Cooke JP. Genetics of peripheral artery disease. Circulation 2012; 125:3220.

12. Rahman MM, Laher I. Structural and functional alteration of blood vessels caused by cigarette smoking: an overview of molecular mechanisms. Curr Vasc Pharmacol 2007; 5:276.

13. Lu L, Mackay DF, Pell JP. Meta-analysis of the association between cigarette smoking and peripheral arterial disease. Heart 2014; 100:414.

14. Meijer WT, Hoes AW, Rutgers D, et al. Peripheral arterial disease in the elderly: The Rotterdam Study. Arterioscler Thromb Vasc Biol 1998; 18:185.

15. Eldrup-Jorgensen J, Flanigan DP, Brace L, et al. Hypercoagulable states and lower limb ischemia in young adults. J Vasc Surg 1989; 9:334.

16. Jude EB, Oyibo SO, Chalmers N, Boulton AJ. Peripheral arterial disease in diabetic and nondiabetic patients: a comparison of severity and outcome. Diabetes Care 2001; 24:1433.

17. Criqui M, Matsushita K, Aboyans V, Hess C, Hicks K, Kwan T, & et al. (2021). Lower Extremity Peripheral Artery Disease: Contemporary Epidemiology, Management Gaps, and Future Directions - A Scientific Statement From the American Heart Association. American Heart Association, Inc - Journal.

18. Fowkes F, Aboyans V, Fowkes Freya, McDermott M, Sampson U, & Criqui M. (2016). Peripheral artery disease: epidemiology and global perspectives. Nature Reviews - Cardiology 14, pages156-170 (2017).

19. Gerhard H, Gornik HL, Barrett C, Barshes NR, Corriere MA, Drachman DE, & et al. (2016). 2016 AHA/ACC Guideline on the Management of Patients With Lower Extremity Peripheral Artery Disease: A Report of the American College of Cardiology/American Heart Association Task Force on Clinical Practice Guidelines. Circulation. 2017;135(12):e726. .

20. McGee SR, Boyko EJ. Physical examination and chronic lower-extremity ischemia: a critical review. Arch Intern Med 1998; 158:1357.

21. Hennion D, & Siano K. (2013). Diagnosis and Treatment of Peripheral Arterial Disease. American Academy of Family Physicians.

22. Hirsch AT, Criqui MH, Treat-Jacobson D, Regensteiner JG, Creager MA, Olin JW, & et al. (2001). Peripheral arterial disease detection, awareness, and treatment in primary care. JAMA. 2001;286(11):1317. .

23. Iftikhar J, Kullo, M.D, & Rooke T. (2016). Peripheral Artery Disease. N Engl J Med 2016.

24. Gerhard-Herman MD, Gornik HL, Barrett C, et al. 2016 AHA/ACC Guideline on the Management of Patients With Lower Extremity Peripheral Artery Disease: A Report of the American College of Cardiology/American Heart Association Task Force on Clinical Practice Guidelines. Circulation 2017; 135:e726.

25. Layden J, Michaels J, Bermingham S, et al. Diagnosis and management of lower limb peripheral arterial disease: summary of NICE guidance. BMJ 2012; 345:e4947.

26. van Zitteren M, Vriens PW, Heyligers JM, et al. Self-reported symptoms on questionnaires and anatomic lesions on duplex ultrasound examinations in patients with peripheral arterial disease. J Vasc Surg 2012; 55:1025.

27. Layden J, Michaels J, Bermingham S, & Higgins B. (2012). Diagnosis and management of lower limb peripheral arterial disease: summary of NICE guidance. BMJ. 2012;345:e4947.

28. McGee SR, & Boyko EJ (1998). Physical examination and chronic lower-extremity ischemia: a critical review. JAMA - Arch Intern Med. 1998;158(12):1357-136.

29. Peach G, Griffin M, Jones KG, Thompson MM, & Hinchliffe RJ (2012). Diagnosis and management of peripheral arterial disease. BMJ 2012;345:e5208.

30. van Reijen NS, Ponchant K, Ubbink DT, Koelemay MJW. Editor's Choice - The Prognostic Value of the WIFI Classification in Patients with Chronic Limb Threatening Ischaemia: A Systematic Review and Meta-Analysis. Eur J Vasc Endovasc Surg 2019; 58:362.

31. Mills JL Sr, Conte MS, Armstrong DG, et al. The Society for Vascular Surgery Lower Extremity Threatened Limb Classification System: risk stratification based on wound, ischemia, and foot infection (WIfI). J Vasc Surg 2014; 59:220.

32. Serrano F, & Conejero A. (2007). Peripheral Artery Disease: Pathophysiology, Diagnosis, and Treatment. Revista Española Cardiología.

33. Signorelli S, Marino E, Scuto S, & Di Raimondo D. (2020). Pathophysiology of Peripheral Arterial Disease (PAD): A Review on Oxidative Disorders. International Journal of Molecular Sciences,2020, 21, 4393.

34. Ulrich F, Sigrid N, & Belch J. (2019). Guideline on peripheral arterial disease. European Journal of Vascular Medicine, 10-35.

35. Elfghi M, Jordan F, Dunne D, Gibson I, Jones J, et al (2021). The effect of lifestyle and risk factor modification on occlusive peripheral arterial disease outcomes: standard healthcare vs structured programme-for a randomised controlled trial protocol. Elfghi et al. Trials (2021) 22:138.

36. Golledge J, Moxon JV, Rowbotham S, et al. Risk of major amputation in patients with intermittent claudication undergoing early revascularization. Br J Surg 2018; 105:699.

37. Murphy TP, Cutlip DE, Regensteiner JG, et al. Supervised exercise, stent revascularization, or medical therapy for claudication due to aortoiliac peripheral artery disease: the CLEVER study. J Am Coll Cardiol 2015; 65:999.

38. Golledge J (2022). Update on the pathophysiology and medical treatment of peripheral artery disease. Nature Reviews Cardiology

39. Khan S, Cleanthis M, Smout J, Flather M, Stansby G. (2005). Life-style Modification in Peripheral Arterial Disease. Eur J Vasc Endovasc Surg 29, 2-9 (2005).

40. Creasy TS, McMillan PJ, Fletcher EW, et al. Is percutaneous transluminal angioplasty better than exercise for claudication? Preliminary results from a prospective randomised trial. Eur J Vasc Surg 1990; 4:135.

41. Fakhry F, Fokkenrood HJ, Spronk S, et al. Endovascular revascularisation versus conservative management for intermittent claudication. Cochrane Database Syst Rev 2018; 3:CD010512.

42. Pulli R, Dorigo W, Fargion A, et al. Early and long-term comparison of endovascular treatment of iliac artery occlusions and stenosis. J Vasc Surg 2011; 53:92.

43. Leville CD, Kashyap VS, Clair DG, et al. Endovascular management of iliac artery occlusions: extending treatment to TransAtlantic Inter-Society Consensus class C and D patients. J Vasc Surg 2006; 43:32.

44. Graham H, Khendi T, Solaru W. (2020) Evidence-Based Medical Management of Peripheral Artery Disease. Arterioscler Thromb Vasc Biol. 2020;40:541-553.

45. Biscetti F, Nardella E, Rando M, Cecchini A, Gasbarrini A, et al. (2021) Outcomes of Lower Extremity Endovascular Revascularization: Potential Predictors and Prevention Strategies. Int. J. Mol. Sci. 2021

46. Kazakov, Y. Lukin, I. Sokolova, N. Ivanova, O. Bakulina, A. (2019). Outcomes of revascularizing operations on lower-limb arteries in patients with critical ischaemia andmultifocal atherosclerosis. Angiol Sosud Khir. 2019;25(3):114-121.doi: 10.33529/ANGIO2019317.

47. Bastos, F. Menyhei, G. Jongkind, V. Svetlikov, A. European Society for Vascular Surgery (ESVS) 2020 Clinical Practice Guidelines on the Management of Acute Limb Ischaemia.

48. Bonaca, M. Hamburg, N. Creager, M. (2021). Contemporary Medical Management of Peripheral Artery Disease. Circ Res. 2021 Jun 11;128(12):1868-1884. doi: 10.1161/CIRCRESAHA.121.318258. Epub 2021 Jun 10.

49. Arias F, Benalcázar S, Bustamante B, Esparza J, et al. (2022). Diagnosis and treatment of peripheral vascular disease. Bibliographic review. Revista Angiología 00421 / http://dx.doi.org/10.20960/angiologia.00421

CONTENTS

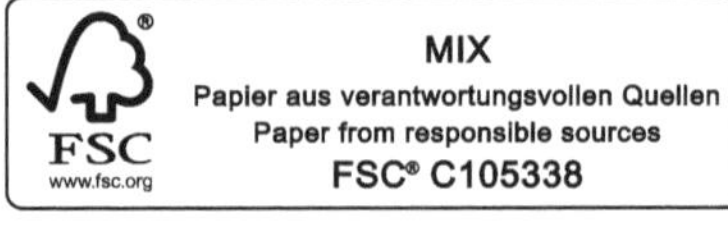

Printed by Books on Demand GmbH, Norderstedt / Germany